Starch-Based Diet

A Beginner's Overview, Review, and Commentary with Recipes

mf

copyright © 2023 Tyler Spellmann

All rights reserved No part of this book may be reproduced, or stored in a retrieval system, or transmitted in any form or by any means, electronic, mechanical, photocopying, recording, or otherwise, without express written permission of the publisher.

Disclaimer

By reading this disclaimer, you are accepting the terms of the disclaimer in full. If you disagree with this disclaimer, please do not read the guide.

All of the content within this guide is provided for informational and educational purposes only, and should not be accepted as independent medical or other professional advice. The author is not a doctor, physician, nurse, mental health provider, or registered nutritionist/dietician. Therefore, using and reading this guide does not establish any form of a physician-patient relationship.

Always consult with a physician or another qualified health provider with any issues or questions you might have regarding any sort of medical condition. Do not ever disregard any qualified professional medical advice or delay seeking that advice because of anything you have read in this guide. The information in this guide is not intended to be any sort of medical advice and should not be used in lieu of any medical advice by a licensed and qualified medical professional.

The information in this guide has been compiled from a variety of known sources. However, the author cannot attest to or guarantee the accuracy of each source and thus should not be held liable for any errors or omissions.

You acknowledge that the publisher of this guide will not be held liable for any loss or damage of any kind incurred as a result of this guide or the reliance on any information provided within this guide. You acknowledge and agree that you assume all risk and responsibility for any action you undertake in response to the information in this guide.

Using this guide does not guarantee any particular result (e.g., weight loss or a cure). By reading this guide, you acknowledge that there are no guarantees to any specific outcome or results you can expect.

All product names, diet plans, or names used in this guide are for identification purposes only and are the property of their respective owners. The use of these names does not imply endorsement. All other trademarks cited herein are the property of their respective owners.

Where applicable, this guide is not intended to be a substitute for the original work of this diet plan and is, at most, a supplement to the original work for this diet plan and never a direct substitute. This guide is a personal expression of the facts of that diet plan.

Where applicable, persons shown in the cover images are stock photography models and the publisher has obtained the rights to use the images through license agreements with third-party stock image companies.

Table of Contents

Introduction — 7
Background and Overview of the Starch-Based Diet — 10
    Diet Composition — 11
    On Weight Loss — 12
    Key Health Benefits of a Starch-Based Diet — 12
    Diet Characteristics — 13
    Challenges and Adaptations — 13
The Development of the Starch-Based Diet Plan — 15
    The Terrifying Change in Diet — 15
    Development of the Starch-Based Diet Plan — 16
    Philosophy and Reception — 17
    Overview of the Starch-Based Diet According to Dr. McDougall — 17
    On Weight Loss and Starchy Foods — 18
    Promised Benefits — 20
The Health Benefits of a Starch-Based Diet — 21
    Health Benefits: Weight Loss and Prevention of Illnesses — 22
    The Success of the Starch-Based Diet Program — 23
Weighing the Pros and Cons — 24
    Pros of the Starch-Based Diet: — 24
    Cons of the Starch-Based Diet: — 25
    Difficulty in Implementation — 25
    Navigating Challenges — 25
Starchy Food Guide — 27
    Nutrition Guide — 28
    Foods to Avoid — 31
5 Step-by-Step Guide to Getting Started with Starch-Based Diet — 33
    Step 1: Understand the Basics of a Starch-Based Diet — 33

Step 2: Plan Your Meals	35
Step 3: Stock Your Kitchen	37
Step 4: Prepare and Enjoy Your Meals	39
Step 5: Monitor Your Progress and Adjust as Needed	42
Starch-Based Diet Recipes	**45**
Caribbean Style Rice	46
Rice Congee	48
Garlic Vegetables Fried Rice	50
Peanut Butter Noodles	52
Kimchi Fried Rice	54
Korean Bean Sprout Salad	56
Bacon and Potato Salad	58
Roasted Vegetables	60
Vegan Corn and Potato Chowder	62
Apple and Onion Mix	64
Mixed Veggie Fried Rice	66
Vegan Potato Curry in Instapot	69
Sweet Potato and Ginger	71
Rice and Peas	74
Baked Potato	76
Conclusion	**78**
FAQs	**80**
References and Helpful Links	**83**

Introduction

In recent years, the conversation around healthy eating and sustainable diets has taken center stage in both wellness communities and environmental discussions. Amidst the myriad of dietary options and philosophies, one approach that has quietly but steadily gained traction is the starch-based diet. This diet, characterized by its focus on whole, plant-based foods with starches at its core, offers a refreshing simplicity in an often overly complicated nutritional landscape.

For those seeking a dietary shift that aligns with both health aspirations and ethical considerations, the starch-based diet emerges as a compelling choice. It stands out not only for its nutritional benefits but also for its ease of adoption in daily life. The foundation of this diet rests on foods that have sustained civilizations for millennia, bringing a sense of tradition and time-tested wisdom to our modern plates.

Transitioning to a starch-based diet doesn't mean embarking on a journey of restriction or culinary monotony. On the contrary, it opens the door to a diverse world of flavors and ingredients, redefining what it means to eat healthily.

This diet emphasizes the importance of whole, minimally processed foods, encouraging a reconnection with natural tastes and textures that many of us have lost touch with. By focusing on starch-rich foods, individuals find themselves exploring a variety of grains, legumes, and root vegetables that form the cornerstone of numerous cuisines around the globe.

The beauty of adopting a starch-based diet lies not just in its health implications but also in its accessibility and sustainability. It's a diet that respects the planet as much as it does our bodies, promoting agricultural practices that are more in harmony with the earth's ecosystems.

Moreover, it challenges the myth that healthy eating must come at a premium, proving that nourishment and flavor can come from humble and affordable ingredients. The simplicity of the starch-based diet also makes it incredibly adaptable, fitting into various lifestyles and dietary preferences with ease.

While the journey towards incorporating more starch-based foods into one's diet is personal and unique, the first step is always rooted in curiosity and openness. Whether you're intrigued by the potential health benefits, drawn to the environmental advantages, or simply looking for a way to bring more variety to your meals, exploring the principles of the starch-based diet could be the beginning of a transformative journey.

As we delve deeper into this dietary approach, it becomes clear that what might seem like a small shift in eating habits can indeed have profound impacts on our health, the environment, and even our cultural appreciation of food.

This starch-based diet review will help you discover:

- What a starch-based diet is
- Why it is healthy
- How eating a starch-based diet can help you lose weight
- A 5 Step-by-Step Guide on How to Get Started with Starch-Based Diet
- Whether this type of diet is perfect for you
- How easy it is to prepare this diet with some recommended recipes

Keep reading to learn more about the benefits of a starch-based diet and how it can improve your overall health.

Background and Overview of the Starch-Based Diet

About forty years ago, the starch-based diet plan was recommended by John McDougall, MD when, after some observation of the three generations of his patients, he noticed that the health status of some of his younger patients started to decline.

On the other hand, their older relatives remained healthy and almost disease-free. The first generation were Asian immigrants, who came from China, Japan, and the Philippines. It is well known from then and even until now that the staple foods of Asians are rice and vegetables.

However, as part of their changing lifestyle as immigrants to the United States, the younger generation's diet started to adopt the Western diet, which consisted mainly of meats, dairy, and oily food. There is also the overwhelming presence of junk food in the diet, not just chips and soda, but also food items that are high in preservatives.

Dr. McDougall took note of this lifestyle shift as well as the overwhelming health deterioration of the younger generation of these Asian families. Where the older relatives have longer life spans with more active lifestyles and almost no illnesses, the younger ones have sadly lost those traits and have also seemingly adopted the American health issues as well.

With these observations, the doctor researched more about the type of diet that heavily contains starch—rice and potatoes—to which he learned that previous research mimicked his discovery.

Diet Composition

From this, the starch-based diet was developed. John A. McDougall, MD, emphasized that starches are plant-based and high in fiber and are in fact, healthy. Notable foods that comprised the diet plan were potatoes, grains, and legumes. The starch-based diet, which is vegan by nature, advocates the concept of losing weight by putting starch-rich plant foods as the main component of your meal.

Dr. McDougall said that this diet must consist of the following composition: starch at 70%, vegetable at 20%, and fruit at 10%. Any meat, dairy, and fat products must be avoided.

The normal American diet would usually be composed of more meat and dairy products and fewer starch, fruits, and vegetables. This is evident in how the United States continues to be among the top meat-eaters in the world, with a daily diet that almost always includes burgers, chicken, and steak.

The starch-based diet, on the other hand, puts more starch-based food, some fruits, vegetables, and little to no meat and dairy. The diet does not just remove animal products, including dairy, but also gets rid of oils, including vegetable oils, sugar, and processed food.

On Weight Loss

Regarding its weight loss efficacy, the starch-based diet focuses on the concept that losing weight involves consuming mainly complex carbohydrates. This is because health and diet experts say complex carbohydrates are essential parts of a healthy balanced diet.

They are rich in dietary fiber, vitamin B, and minerals, elements that the human body needs in regulating blood sugar levels and promotion of digestive health that is why they are important in a healthy starch-based diet. Complex carbohydrates can be found generally in whole grains. Other sources include brown or red rice, barley, oats, vegetables rich in starch, legumes, sweet potatoes, and a lot more.

Key Health Benefits of a Starch-Based Diet

Adopting a starch-based diet offers significant health advantages, primarily highlighted by two major benefits:

Reduced Risk of Diabetes

A key advantage of a starch-based, vegan diet is its potential to lower the risk of developing diabetes. This benefit is largely attributed to the high fiber content found in plant-based foods. Fiber plays a crucial role in managing and stabilizing blood sugar levels, thus offering protection against diabetes.

Enhanced Digestive Health

Another significant benefit is improved digestion. The abundance of fiber in a starch-based diet supports digestive health by maintaining the health of colon cells and ensuring the smooth operation of the digestive tract. This helps prevent blockages and keeps the system clean.

Diet Characteristics

The diet is predominantly plant-based, focusing on fiber-rich foods, which appeal to vegans and anyone looking to improve their health through diet.

It advocates for the elimination of meat, dairy, and added sugars—the latter being linked to numerous chronic diseases and considered one of the most harmful food ingredients.

Challenges and Adaptations

Adherents may face challenges such as eliminating favorite foods including meats, sugary snacks like donuts and chocolates, and even common additives like olive oil in salads.

Despite these challenges, the diet offers flexibility, allowing for meals and snacks anytime—as long as they are starch-based and low in fat. This includes options for snacks and desserts within the dietary guidelines.

While transitioning to a starch-based diet requires time, effort, dedication, and consistency, the health benefits can be substantial. According to Dr. McDougall's research and testimonials from individuals who have adopted this diet, the improvements in health and well-being significantly outweigh the initial difficulties. This diet not only promotes better health outcomes but also encourages a more mindful and sustainable way of eating.

The Development of the Starch-Based Diet Plan

Studies have shown how nutrition and health are closely linked with the emergence of various new diseases over the past century. Because of some drastic changes in diet, eating habits, and lifestyle, specifically the marked nutrient deficiencies in man's diet, there has been a steadily observed rise in chronic diet-related diseases.

One of the country's nutrition experts who has been leading the search for the diet plan to avert the continuous rise of chronic diseases that may be linked to what is considered a toxic diet discovered in the 1970s what could now be considered the return of human civilization to the food that has made it survive throughout these centuries.

The Terrifying Change in Diet

In the 1970s, while working on a Hawaiian sugar plantation, Dr. John McDougall observed a concerning trend among the island's growing Asian immigrant population. Their health deteriorated as they shifted away from their traditional diets towards Western eating habits.

Here are the key points from Dr. McDougall's observations and subsequent dietary plan:

Observation of Health Decline

Dr. McDougall noticed a health decline among Asian immigrants who started consuming more meat, processed foods cooked in oil, increased dairy, and high levels of fat and sugar.

Traditional Diet

Traditionally, these populations relied on staples like starch-rich rice and potatoes.

Dietary Shift and Its Impact

The adoption of a Western diet marked by high meat, dairy, and processed food intake was linked to the observed health issues.

Development of the Starch-Based Diet Plan

To counteract this decline in health, Dr. McDougall formulated a diet plan centered on the traditional staple foods:

- Elimination of fish, meat, eggs, and dairy products
- Increased consumption of vegetables, fruits, and starch-rich foods such as rice, potatoes, barley, and sweet potatoes.
- Removal of oil in cooking and reduction of sugar and salt intake.

Philosophy and Reception

Dr. McDougall advocates that humans are naturally inclined to eat starch-based diets, suggesting that political and economic changes have negatively impacted our diet, leading to nutrient deficiencies. His diet plan, being natural and plant-based, has gained popularity, especially among vegans.

Dr. McDougall's work highlights the significant impact of diet on health and proposes a return to more traditional, starch-based eating habits to improve well-being.

Overview of the Starch-Based Diet According to Dr. McDougall

Dr. McDougall's "Starch Solution" emphasizes a diet that is a nod to ancient human eating habits, focusing on consuming more carbohydrates than proteins and fats. This diet includes a variety of food groups but prioritizes starch-rich foods.

Key Aspects of the Starch-Based Diet

- *Inclusion of Various Food Groups*: While the diet is centered around starch, it also encourages the consumption of fruits, vegetables, small servings of nuts, edible seeds, soy, various food products, and some refined grains.
- *Elimination of Traditional Protein Sources*: The diet excludes meat, poultry, eggs, seafood, dairy products, and processed or prepackaged foods.

- ***No Caloric Restriction***: There is no limit on the number of calories. Eating when hungry is encouraged, even if it's soon after the last meal.

Core Components of the Starch-Based Diet

The diet is structured around three main groups of starches:

- ***Grains***: Including rice, oats, wheat, corn, and millet, among others.
- ***Legumes***: Encompassing all kinds of beans (lima, soybeans, kidney beans, chickpeas, mung, etc.), peas (black-eyed, yellow, garden sweet, spring, sugar snap, snowbird, etc.), and peanuts (to be consumed minimally).
- ***Starchy Vegetables***: Such as sweet potatoes, taro, white potatoes, yam, winter squash, pumpkin, and more.

On Weight Loss and Starchy Foods

When aiming for weight loss with a starch-based diet, the approach emphasizes a balanced intake of starchy and non-starchy vegetables, with a minimal addition of fruits. The key points of this diet plan for effective weight loss include:

Balanced Vegetable Intake

Equal amounts of starchy and non-starchy vegetables are recommended to leverage their low-calorie benefits, essential for creating a calorie deficit needed for weight loss.

Minimal Fruit Addition

While fruits are included, their quantities should be limited to avoid excess sugar intake.

Watch Out for Additives

It's crucial to monitor the use of food condiments and additives, ensuring they are low in fat, sugar, and salt to maintain the diet's effectiveness.

Flexible Eating Schedule

Unlike other diets, there is no strict rule on the quantity or frequency of meals. The focus is on eating the right foods, not how much or how often, allowing for eating whenever hunger strikes without deprivation.

Elimination of Oil

One of the major challenges is avoiding oil in food preparation, a common staple in cooking.

Avoidance of Meat, Dairy, and Fat

Ensuring minimal to no consumption of meat, dairy, and fats is vital, as their combination with carbohydrates can lead to health issues and weight gain.

Promised Benefits

Adherents report significant weight loss, increased energy, and a lower risk of chronic diseases like type-2 diabetes and heart disease when the diet is followed rigorously.

This diet stands out for its focus on what to eat rather than how much, offering a flexible approach that doesn't compromise the joy of eating while aiming for weight loss and improved health outcomes.

The Health Benefits of a Starch-Based Diet

Studies continue to show that more and more people are attempting to lose weight. Over time, changes in diet, the introduction of various ways to prepare and cook food, and the use of a lot of both natural and artificial additives have contributed to the kind of weight and health problems that a lot of people around the world are going through now.

Obesity has been considered a global pandemic. This global nutritional revolution coupled with an increasingly sedentary lifestyle is seen as the culprit. A study shows that by about 2030, there will be 2.16 billion obese adults in the world. To provide some perspective, that is around 25% of the entire world's population. Undeniably, diet change is imperative, whether it is to lose weight and/or for health reasons.

According to Dr. John McDougall, the starch-based diet is the most ideal food for humans, as evidenced by how he has seen it in the people he has treated. He says it is also nature's best-kept secret to losing weight, to providing improved overall well-being.

Health Benefits: Weight Loss and Prevention of Illnesses

The starch-based diet, while not directly linked to fat loss, emphasizes a significant reduction or complete elimination of animal fats and processed foods, which are primary sources of salt, saturated fat, and sugar—key contributors to weight gain.

The diet focuses on plant-based foods, particularly those containing "resistant starch," such as potatoes, rye bread, oatmeal, and bananas, known for their lower calorie content.

Here are the organized key points regarding the health benefits, including weight loss and illness prevention, associated with the starch-based diet:

Reduction of Animal Fats and Processed Foods: Essential for cutting back on salt, saturated fat, and sugar.

Focus on Resistant Starches: Foods like potatoes, rye bread, oatmeal, and bananas help reduce hunger, cut down food cravings, and more effectively burn fats. These starches also aid in fat burning by the liver.

Personal Health Journey of Dr. McDougall: Suffered from frequent illnesses and obesity due to a diet rich in meat and processed foods. Experienced a stroke, which he later attributed to his animal-based diet.

Observations on Asian Immigrants: Noted their health decline upon shifting from a starch-rich diet to one high in meat and dairy, correlating with an increase in diseases such as diabetes, heart disease, arthritis, and cancer.

Health and Diet Studies: Research supports that many modern illnesses are linked to diet and lifestyle choices.

The Success of the Starch-Based Diet Program

- Significant weight loss among participants.
- Reduction in cholesterol levels.
- Prevention or mitigation of the effects of existing illnesses.

The starch-based diet, centered on plant-based and resistant starch foods, has shown promising results in preventing diseases and reversing their effects, alongside aiding in weight loss and improving overall health. It raises the question of its applicability for everyone and whether it can be universally recommended.

Weighing the Pros and Cons

The starch-based diet, as advocated by Dr. McDougall, emphasizes the natural inclination of humans towards consuming starch-rich, plant-based foods while eliminating meat and dairy products.

This approach is touted for its numerous health benefits, including weight loss and disease prevention. However, it's essential to consider both the advantages and potential drawbacks before adopting this diet fully.

Here's a more organized summary of the key points:

Pros of the Starch-Based Diet:

- *Natural and Healthy*: Dr. McDougall asserts that humans are naturally inclined to consume a starch-rich diet, which can significantly improve one's health status and overall well-being.
- *Weight Loss and Disease Prevention*: The diet has been linked to considerable weight loss, lower cholesterol levels, and the prevention or mitigation of certain diseases.

Cons of the Starch-Based Diet:

- *Low in Fat*: Lacey Bourassa notes that the diet is low in fat, raising concerns about the absorption of fat-soluble vitamins (A, K, E, D) and the importance of omega fatty acids found in fish oil for cell membrane structure. However, Dr. McDougall contends that the fats present in starches and vegetables are sufficient for the body's needs.

Difficulty in Implementation

The diet requires time and effort to find and prepare the recommended foods, which might be challenging for individuals with busy schedules.

Dining out can be problematic since not all establishments offer suitable options, and there's a risk of consuming foods cooked with oil or dairy products.

Navigating Challenges

- *Commitment Is Key*: Adopting this diet demands dedication, time, effort, and sometimes an increased budget. It's crucial to plan meals carefully, especially when eating outside, to stay within the diet's guidelines.
- *Resilience*: Occasional lapses are understandable, given the diet's complexity. The important thing is to

quickly realign with the diet's principles and continue striving towards one's health goals.

While the starch-based diet presents several health benefits and aligns with sustainable, earth-friendly practices, potential participants must weigh these advantages against the challenges of low dietary fat and the practical difficulties of adhering to the diet.

Success relies on commitment, careful planning, and a willingness to embrace a significant lifestyle change, alongside regular exercise and healthy habits.

Starchy Food Guide

If you're considering adopting a starch-based diet, there's a wide array of starchy foods available that can serve as excellent energy sources. Here's a guide to various types of starchy foods that are not only nutritious but also versatile in meal planning.

Bread

A staple source of starch and fiber, especially for those without wheat allergies or intolerances. Opt for varieties like brown, granary, seeded, and wholemeal bread, which are packed with fiber, minerals, and vitamins B and E. While white bread can also be part of your diet, aim for options that are high in fiber.

Cereals

Consuming wholegrain cereal products daily can provide you with essential nutrients such as fiber, iron, protein, and B vitamins. These include barley, corn, couscous, oats, rice, rye, tapioca, and wheat, making them ideal choices for a nutritious breakfast.

Grains and Rice

Similar to cereal products, grains and rice are rich in fiber, protein, and B vitamins, while being low in fat. They're excellent energy sources. You can choose from a variety of grains like arborio, basmati, brown, long and short grains, quick-cook, and wild rice, as well as bulgur and couscous.

Pasta

For a good intake of iron and vitamin B, consider wholegrain and wholewheat pasta. Its high fiber content means digestion is slower, helping you feel fuller for longer periods.

Potatoes

Well-known for their starchy content, potatoes, particularly when eaten with their skin, are rich in carbohydrates, fiber, potassium, and B vitamins. They're a fantastic source of energy, low in calories and fat.

Incorporating these starchy foods into your diet can provide the necessary nutrients to fuel your body efficiently. They also offer the added benefit of being low in calories and fat, making them ideal for a healthy, balanced diet.

Nutrition Guide

Starchy foods are important sources of nutrition in one's regular meals and are considered one of the key food groups.

It's recommended that a third of a regular diet should have about starchy food items.

Normally, there are five food groups as recommended by USDA (US Department of Agriculture), as symbolized by the MyPlate icon—there's dairy, fruits, grains, protein foods, and vegetables. As for the Eatwell Guide provided by the Irish government, the five food groups consisted of the following:

- protein-rich products including beans, eggs, fish, meat
- dairy and the likes
- fruit and vegetables
- spreads and unsaturated oils
- starchy carbohydrates like bread, pasta, potatoes, and rice

All these starchy foods are great sources of several nutrients and vitamins, and here are as follows:

Fiber

As we all know, fiber keeps our digestive systems healthy and assists in weight loss. It's a type of carbohydrate that the body consumes but cannot digest. One of its main roles is to make sure that the blood sugar is okay. Fiber also helps keep the body feeling full.

It's important to know the two types of fiber—soluble and insoluble.

Soluble fiber assists in the reduction of cholesterol in the blood as well as glucose levels. It's called as such because it dissolves in water.

Some examples of good sources of soluble fibers are as follows: beans, blueberries, chia seeds, lentils, nuts, oats, and pulses.

From its name itself, insoluble fiber does not dissolve in water. However, it aids the food so it can get through the body's digestive system. With this, you can rely on a regular bowel movement and don't have to worry about constipation.

The following are good sources of insoluble fibers: almonds, apples (with skin), brown rice, kale, legumes, pears (with skin), quinoa, seeds, walnuts, wheat bran, and other whole wheat products like pasta. Wholegrain products such as bread, brown rice, and cereals.

B vitamins

There are many benefits provided by B vitamins that affect digestion, brain function, and cardiovascular health, to name a few. Starchy foods may give thiamin or vitamin B1, which is essential in making sure that the energy provided by the carbohydrates we consume is being used. Vitamin B9 or folate is great at making sure that the red blood cells are formed healthily, as well as the growth and function of the cells in the body.

Calcium

Starchy foods are also rich in calcium, which is a nutrient responsible for keeping the body's bones and teeth healthy. It also helps the muscles and nerves to function well.

Iron

Iron-rich foods like starchy foods are important to help mainly with the production of hemoglobin, or the protein found in the red blood cells, which carry the oxygen around the body. It's also important for the immune system and normal brain function, which helps in enhancing memory and sports performance.

Foods to Avoid

In a starch-based diet, especially if you're aiming for weight loss or maintaining a healthy lifestyle, it's advisable to avoid certain foods that might hinder your goals. These include:

- *Potato Chips*: High in fat, additives, and salt, potato chips are calorie-dense with little nutritional value.
- *Refined Starches*: Foods made from refined grains, such as white bread, white rice, and other processed foods, lack essential nutrients, fiber, vitamins, and minerals.
- *Cornmeal and Millet Flour*: When highly processed, these can be high in starch but low in nutritional value.

- ***High-Starch Processed Foods***: This includes pretzels, pasta, and bread made from refined flour, which can contribute to blood sugar spikes without providing sufficient nutrients or satiety.
- ***Starchy Vegetables (in excess)***: While not inherently bad, consuming starchy vegetables like potatoes in excessive amounts, especially when fried or prepared with unhealthy fats, can be counterproductive.
- ***Processed Foods High in Starch***: Many packaged snacks, ready-to-eat meals, and fast food items use refined starches and should be consumed minimally.

Focusing on whole, minimally processed starchy foods like whole grains, legumes, and root vegetables can help ensure you're getting the nutrients your body needs while adhering to a starch-based diet.

5 Step-by-Step Guide to Getting Started with Starch-Based Diet

Transitioning to a starch-based diet can be a transformative journey for your health, environment, and taste buds. A starch-based diet emphasizes whole, plant-based foods with starches like potatoes, rice, and beans as the cornerstone of your meals. If you're ready to embrace this lifestyle, here's a comprehensive five-step guide to get you started.

Step 1: Understand the Basics of a Starch-Based Diet

To embark on a starch-based diet effectively, it's essential to delve deep into its foundational principles and the significant nutritional advantages it offers. This diet emphasizes:

- *Whole, Unprocessed, or Minimally Processed Starches*: Central to this diet, these foods serve as the primary energy source and are pivotal for maintaining satiety and stabilizing blood sugar levels.

- *Vegetables and Fruits*: These are integral for adding diversity in flavor, texture, and, most importantly, a wide array of nutrients to the diet.

Key Nutritional Benefits:
- *Complex Carbohydrates*: The backbone of this diet, complex carbs provide a gradual energy release, which is beneficial for blood sugar control and sustained energy levels throughout the day.
- *Dietary Fiber*: High fiber content from these foods aids in digestion, promotes a healthy gut microbiome and has been linked to a reduced risk of several chronic diseases.
- *Vitamins and Minerals*: A broad spectrum of essential nutrients supports various bodily functions—ranging from immune system health to bone strength and neurological function.
- *Antioxidants*: Foods rich in antioxidants help combat oxidative stress and inflammation, contributing to disease prevention and overall well-being.

Staples of a Starch-Based Diet:
- *Potatoes and Sweet Potatoes*: Not just rich in carbohydrates but also a good source of vitamin C, potassium, and dietary fiber.

- *Corn, Peas, Beans, and Lentils*: Besides being hearty sources of protein, these legumes are loaded with iron, zinc, and folate, essential for various bodily functions.
- *Whole Grains and Whole Grain Products*: These include quinoa, brown rice, oats, and barley, which are not only versatile but packed with nutrients.

Understanding these principles and the nutritional powerhouse that a starch-based diet can be is crucial for anyone looking to adopt this healthy eating pattern. It's not merely about choosing specific types of foods but appreciating their role in promoting health and preventing disease. By centering your diet around these staples, you're not only nourishing your body with what it needs but also embracing a lifestyle that prioritizes long-term health and vitality.

Step 2: Plan Your Meals

Now that you have a good understanding of the key components of a starch-based diet, it's time to start planning your meals.

Here are the key steps and considerations for successful meal planning on a starch-based diet:

- *Explore Resources*: Dive into the vast array of online content, cookbooks, and community forums focused on plant-based and vegan lifestyles. These platforms offer valuable recipe ideas, practical tips, and support that align with starch-based dietary principles emphasizing minimally processed, whole, plant-derived foods.

Aim for Variety

- *Starches*: Incorporate a diverse selection of starches such as potatoes, sweet potatoes, and whole grains (e.g., brown rice, quinoa, whole wheat pasta) to form the base of your meals.
- *Legumes*: Add beans, lentils, and chickpeas for their protein, fiber, and nutrient content.
- *Vegetables*: Ensure meals are colorful and nutrient-dense by including a wide range of vegetables, from leafy greens to root varieties.
- *Fruits*: Use fruits as snacks or dessert options for a natural sweetness and nutritional boost.
- *Consider Snacks*: Choose whole, nutrient-rich snacks like fresh fruits, vegetable sticks with hummus, air-popped popcorn, and whole-grain crackers to maintain energy levels between meals.
- *Stay Hydrated*: Emphasize the importance of hydration by including ample fluids such as water, herbal teas, and infused waters in your daily intake, avoiding added calories or sugars.

By dedicating time to thoughtful meal planning, you're more likely to adhere to a starch-based diet successfully, enjoying a variety of nutritious and appealing meals that cater to your health objectives. The ultimate aim of meal planning is not only to meet dietary guidelines but also to relish in satisfying, wholesome food that energizes your body and pleases your palate.

Step 3: Stock Your Kitchen

Once you have your meal plan, it's time to stock your kitchen. Transitioning to a starch-based diet not only involves changing your eating habits but also transforming your kitchen into a space that supports your new lifestyle.

Here's how to effectively stock your kitchen:

Purge Unwanted Items:

Begin by removing highly processed foods, meats, dairy products, and items high in refined sugars and fats from your pantry and fridge. This reduces temptation and makes room for healthier options.

Consider donating unopened, non-perishable items to local food banks or sharing with friends and family.

Plan Your Shopping Trip:

Create a shopping list based on your weekly meal plan. This ensures you purchase everything you need, avoiding multiple trips to the store and impulse buys.

Prioritize whole, unprocessed ingredients to form the foundation of your diet.

Stocking Up

- *Whole Grains and Legumes*: Utilize the bulk sections for items like rice, quinoa, oats, lentils, and beans. Buying in bulk can be more cost-effective and allows you to purchase the exact amount you need, reducing waste.
- *Vegetables and Fruits*: Opt for a variety of fresh produce. If fresh options are limited or expensive, frozen vegetables and fruits are a nutritious and budget-friendly alternative.
- *Spices and Herbs*: These are crucial for adding depth and flavor to your meals without relying on added fats or sugars. Build a diverse spice cabinet to keep your meals exciting.
- *Nuts and Seeds*: While to be used sparingly, nuts and seeds are great for adding crunch and nutrients to dishes. Look for raw or dry-roasted varieties without added oils or salts.
- *Healthy Fats*: Sources like avocados, olives, and small amounts of nuts and seeds. Select heart-healthy oils, such as olive oil, for cooking when necessary.

Organizational Tips

Once home, organize your purchases for easy access. This might mean transferring bulk items into clear, labeled containers for pantry storage.

Keep your fridge and countertops arranged with healthy options in plain sight, encouraging better snack choices.

Ongoing Maintenance

Regularly check your pantry and fridge to restock essentials and experiment with new ingredients to diversify your diet.

Stay informed about seasonal produce to enjoy the freshest options while supporting local agriculture.

By carefully stocking and organizing your kitchen, you create an environment that encourages and simplifies adherence to a starch-based diet. This preparation not only supports your health goals but also enhances your cooking experience, making it easier to maintain this beneficial lifestyle change.

Step 4: Prepare and Enjoy Your Meals

Now that your kitchen is fully stocked and ready to support your starch-based diet, it's time to embark on the exciting journey of meal preparation. If you're navigating the kitchen with fresh eyes or experimenting with these types of ingredients for the first time.

Here's how to approach this new culinary adventure:

Embrace Simplicity:

- *Start with Basic Recipes*: There's no pressure to whip up complex gourmet meals right away. Begin your cooking journey with simple recipes that don't require extensive cooking skills or hard-to-find ingredients. These dishes can be both deeply satisfying and surprisingly easy to make.
- *Appreciate the Flavors*: Even the simplest dishes can be rich in flavor. Discover the joy in the natural taste of whole foods, enhanced with just a few herbs or spices.

Plan meal preparation with Batch Cooking:

- *Cook in Bulk*: Save precious time during your busy week by batch-cooking staple ingredients. Grains like rice, legumes such as beans, and versatile veggies like potatoes can be cooked in larger quantities and stored for later use.
- *Store Smartly*: Keep these cooked staples in clear, labeled containers in your refrigerator. This not only makes it easier to see what you have on hand but also streamlines the meal preparation process when time is scarce.

Explore and Experiment:

- *Try New Recipes*: As you gain confidence in your cooking abilities, start branching out by trying new

recipes. This will not only diversify your diet but also introduce you to new flavors and cooking techniques.
- ***Experiment with Flavors***: Don't be afraid to play with different herbs, spices, and seasonings. A dash of creativity can transform even the most basic dishes into something extraordinary.

Enjoy the Culinary Journey:

- ***Discover New Favorites***: Embrace the opportunity to explore various cuisines and ingredients. You'll likely stumble upon new favorite foods and recipes that you'll want to return to time and again.
- ***Relish the Process***: Cooking is more than just a means to an end; it's a rewarding process that allows you to connect with the food you eat. Enjoy the act of preparing your meals, and take pride in the dishes you create.

By starting simple, planning, being willing to experiment, and enjoying the process, you'll find that preparing and enjoying meals on a starch-based diet can be a delightful and enriching experience.

Remember, this journey is about exploring new tastes and textures, nourishing your body with wholesome foods, and discovering the joy and satisfaction that comes from cooking and eating well.

Step 5: Monitor Your Progress and Adjust as Needed

Embarking on a starch-based diet is not just about changing what you eat; it's also about tuning into your body and being responsive to its needs. As you navigate this dietary transition, it's crucial to monitor your progress and make adjustments as necessary.

Here's how to effectively track your journey and ensure your nutritional requirements are being met:

Listen to Your Body:

- *Monitor How You Feel*: Pay close attention to your overall sense of well-being. Note any changes in your energy levels, mood, and physical comfort. Feeling more vibrant and energetic can be a positive sign that your new diet is benefiting you.
- *Watch for Physical Changes*: Keep an eye on any noticeable changes in your body. This might include weight loss, improved skin clarity, or even better digestion. These changes can serve as indicators of the positive impact of your dietary choices.

Track Health Markers:

- *Observe Blood Sugar and Cholesterol Levels*: A starch-based diet may lead to improvements in key health markers, such as blood sugar control and

cholesterol levels. Regularly checking these can provide concrete evidence of the diet's effects on your health.
- *Note Blood Pressure Changes*: If you're monitoring blood pressure, observe any trends that occur after switching to a starch-based diet. Many find that plant-based diets contribute to better blood pressure management.

Consult Healthcare Professionals:
- *Seek Personalized Advice*: If you have existing health concerns or unique dietary needs, consulting with a healthcare professional or a dietitian who has experience with plant-based diets is essential. They can offer tailored advice to ensure your diet is nutritionally balanced.
- *Adjustments May Be Necessary*: Based on professional guidance, you might need to tweak your diet. This could involve incorporating specific supplements, adjusting macronutrient ratios, or focusing on particular nutrients to ensure your body receives everything it needs.

Stay Informed and Flexible:
- **Educate Yourself**: Continuously educate yourself about plant-based nutrition and the latest research.

Knowledge is power, and staying informed will help you make the best decisions for your health.

- **Be Open to Adjustments**: Recognize that dietary needs can evolve. Be prepared to adjust your eating habits as needed to align with your health goals and lifestyle changes.

By closely monitoring your progress and being open to making necessary adjustments, you can optimize the benefits of a starch-based diet. Remember, the goal is not only to adopt healthier eating patterns but also to ensure that those patterns align with your individual health needs and goals. Through mindful observation and possibly professional guidance, you can fine-tune your diet to support your health and well-being fully.

Starch-Based Diet Recipes

Caribbean Style Rice

Ingredients:

- 1 cup brown rice, uncooked
- 2 cups vegetable broth (ensure it's low-sodium and oil-free)
- 1 can (15 oz) black beans, rinsed and drained
- 1 red bell pepper, diced
- 1 yellow bell pepper, diced
- 1 medium onion, diced
- 2 cloves garlic, minced
- 1 cup pineapple, diced (fresh or canned in juice, not syrup)
- 1 teaspoon of powdered cumin
- 1 teaspoon of coriander powder
- 1/2 teaspoon of allspice powder
- 1/4 teaspoon of cayenne pepper powder (adjust according to heat preference)
- 1/2 cup fresh cilantro, chopped
- Juice of 1 lime
- Salt and pepper to taste (optional)

Instructions:

1. In a large pot, bring the vegetable broth to a boil.
2. Add the brown rice, reduce the heat to low, cover, and simmer for about 45 minutes, or until the rice is cooked and all the liquid is absorbed.

3. While the rice is cooking, heat a large, non-stick skillet over medium heat.
4. Add a splash of vegetable broth or water to prevent sticking, then sauté the onion and garlic until translucent, about 3-5 minutes.
5. Add the diced red and yellow bell peppers to the skillet.
6. Continue to cook, stirring occasionally, until the peppers are soft, about 5 more minutes.
7. Once the rice is cooked, fluff it with a fork and add it to the skillet with the vegetables.
8. Add the black beans, pineapple, cumin, coriander, allspice, and cayenne pepper to the skillet. Stir well to combine all the ingredients.
9. Cook the mixture over low heat for another 5-10 minutes, stirring occasionally, to allow the flavors to meld together.
10. Remove from heat and stir in the fresh cilantro and lime juice.
11. Taste and adjust seasoning with salt and pepper if desired.
12. Serve hot as a main dish or a hearty side.
13. This Caribbean-style rice pairs wonderfully with a simple green salad or steamed greens for a complete meal.

Rice Congee

Ingredients:

- 1 cup jasmine rice (or short-grain rice)
- 8 cups water (or vegetable broth for more flavor)
- 1-inch piece of ginger peeled and thinly sliced

Optional toppings:

- Sliced scallions
- Chopped cilantro
- Steamed bok choy or spinach
- Sautéed mushrooms (use water or vegetable broth to sauté)
- Soy sauce or tamari (ensure it's low sodium)
- Chili paste or flakes for heat

Instructions:

1. Rinse the jasmine rice under cold water until the water runs clear. This step is important to remove excess starch and prevent the congee from becoming too thick too quickly.
2. In a large pot, combine the rinsed rice, water (or vegetable broth), and sliced ginger.
3. Bring the mixture to a boil over high heat.
4. Once boiling, reduce the heat to a low simmer and partially cover the pot with a lid.

5. Stir occasionally to prevent the rice from sticking to the bottom of the pot.
6. Simmer for about 1 to 1.5 hours, or until the congee reaches your desired consistency. For a thicker congee, cook longer.
7. For a thinner congee, you may add more water or broth as needed during cooking.
8. After the congee has cooked and reached your desired consistency, remove the ginger slices.
9. Taste the congee and adjust the seasoning as needed.
10. You can add a little bit of salt if necessary, but the optional toppings will also add flavor.
11. Ladle the hot congee into bowls and add your preferred toppings.
12. The beauty of congee is its versatility; you can customize each bowl with different toppings to suit individual tastes.

Garlic Vegetables Fried Rice

Ingredients:

- 4 cups cooked brown rice (preferably cooked a day ahead and chilled)
- 1/2 cup water (for sautéing)
- 6-8 cloves garlic, minced
- 1/2 cup finely diced onion
- 1 cup chopped carrots
- 1 cup frozen peas, thawed
- 1 cup chopped bell peppers (any color)
- 1 cup chopped broccoli florets
- 2-3 tablespoons soy sauce or tamari (low sodium)
- 1 tablespoon grated ginger
- 2 green onions, sliced for garnish
- Black pepper to taste
- Optional: chili flakes for a spicy kick

Instructions:

1. Ensure your brown rice is cooked, ideally a day ahead, and stored in the refrigerator.
2. This helps to firm up the grains and prevents the fried rice from becoming mushy.
3. In a large non-stick skillet or wok, heat 1/4 cup of water over medium heat.
4. Incorporate the chopped garlic and onion, cooking them until they become aromatic and clear.

5. Add more water as needed to prevent sticking.
6. To the skillet, add the carrots, bell peppers, and broccoli.
7. Stir well and cook until the vegetables are tender but still crisp about 5-7 minutes.
8. If the mixture begins to stick, add a little more water.
9. Add the cooked brown rice, thawed peas, grated ginger, and soy sauce or tamari to the skillet.
10. Mix thoroughly to combine all the ingredients.
11. Cook for another 5-10 minutes, stirring frequently to ensure the rice heats through and absorbs the flavors.
12. Once everything is heated through and well combined, remove from heat.
13. Taste and adjust seasoning with black pepper and chili flakes if desired.
14. Garnish with sliced green onions before serving.

Peanut Butter Noodles

Ingredients:

- 8 oz whole wheat or brown rice noodles (for gluten-free option)
- 3 tablespoons natural peanut butter (unsweetened and unsalted)
- 2 tablespoons low-sodium soy sauce or tamari (for a gluten-free option)
- 1 tablespoon maple syrup (instead of refined sugar)
- 1 clove garlic, minced
- 1 teaspoon grated fresh ginger
- 1/2 cup water (to adjust sauce consistency)

Optional for serving:

- Sliced green onions
- Crushed peanuts
- Chili flakes
- Lime wedges

Instructions:

1. Bring a large pot of water to a boil and cook the noodles according to package instructions until al dente.
2. Once cooked, drain and rinse under cold water to stop the cooking process. Set aside.

3. In a bowl, whisk together the peanut butter, soy sauce or tamari, maple syrup, minced garlic, and grated ginger.
4. Gradually add water to the mixture until you achieve a smooth and pourable sauce consistency.
5. Adjust the amount of water depending on how thick or thin you prefer your sauce.
6. In a big mixing bowl, mix the prepared noodles with the peanut sauce until they are uniformly covered.
7. If the noodles have cooled down too much, you can briefly heat them in a pan over medium heat, stirring constantly to prevent sticking.
8. Serve the peanut butter noodles in bowls, garnished with optional toppings such as sliced green onions, crushed peanuts, chili flakes, and lime wedges on the side for an added zesty flavor.

Kimchi Fried Rice

Ingredients:

- 2 cups cooked brown rice (preferably cooked a day ahead and chilled)
- 1 cup vegan kimchi, chopped (ensure it's free from fish sauce)
- 1/4 cup kimchi juice (for flavor)
- 1/2 cup water or vegetable broth (for sautéing)
- 1/2 yellow onion, diced
- 2 green onions, sliced (separate white and green parts)
- 1 carrot, diced
- 1/2 cup frozen peas, thawed
- 2 cloves garlic, minced
- 1 teaspoon grated fresh ginger
- 2 tablespoons soy sauce or tamari (low sodium)
- Optional: Tofu, cubed and baked for a protein boost
- Black pepper to taste

Instructions:

1. Ensure the brown rice is cooked ahead of time and chilled. This helps to prevent the rice from becoming mushy when fried.
2. If adding tofu, pre-bake or prepare it according to your preference before starting with the rice.

3. Warm up 1/4 cup of water or vegetable broth in a spacious non-stick skillet or wok, setting the stove to a medium temperature.
4. Incorporate the chopped yellow onion, the white segments of the green onions, and the carrot, cooking them until they begin to become tender, approximately 5 minutes.
5. Incorporate the chopped garlic and shredded ginger, continuing to cook for an additional minute until the aroma is released.
6. Stir in the chopped kimchi, allowing it to cook for a couple of minutes.
7. Then, add the chilled brown rice, breaking up any clumps.
8. Pour in the kimchi juice and soy sauce or tamari, mixing well to ensure the rice is evenly coated with all the flavors.
9. Add the thawed peas and baked tofu cubes (if using) to the skillet.
10. Stir everything together and let it cook for another 5-7 minutes, or until everything is heated through and combined nicely.
11. If the mixture seems too dry, add a little more water or vegetable broth to reach the desired consistency.
12. Taste and adjust the seasoning with black pepper.
13. Serve hot, garnished with the sliced green parts of the green onions.

Korean Bean Sprout Salad

Ingredients:

- 1 pound mung bean sprouts
- 2 tablespoons water or vegetable broth (for dressing)
- 2 teaspoons low-sodium soy sauce or tamari (gluten-free if necessary)
- 1 clove garlic, minced
- 1 scallion, finely chopped
- 1 tablespoon rice vinegar
- 1 teaspoon ground black pepper

Optional for garnish:

- A sprinkle of toasted sesame seeds (omit if avoiding fats)
- Additional sliced green onions

Instructions:

1. Bring a large pot of water to a boil.
2. Add the bean sprouts and blanch for about 30 seconds to 1 minute, just until they are slightly softened but still crisp.
3. Immediately drain and plunge the bean sprouts into ice water to stop the cooking process and preserve their crunch. Drain well.

4. In a small bowl, whisk together water or vegetable broth, low-sodium soy sauce or tamari, minced garlic, rice vinegar, and black pepper.
5. This creates a flavorful dressing that complements the natural taste of the bean sprouts without the need for oil.
6. In a bowl, mix together the parboiled and strained bean sprouts with the sauce.
7. Add the chopped scallions and toss everything together until the bean sprouts are evenly coated with the dressing.
8. Cover and let the salad chill in the refrigerator for at least 30 minutes.
9. This allows the flavors to meld together.
10. Before serving, give the salad a quick toss.
11. Garnish with toasted sesame seeds and additional sliced green onions, if desired.
12. Serve chilled as a refreshing side dish.

Bacon and Potato Salad

Ingredients:

- 2 pounds small red or yellow potatoes, cut into bite-sized pieces
- 1/4 cup water or vegetable broth (for sautéing and dressing)
- 1/2 cup unsweetened, unflavored plant-based yogurt (soy, almond, or coconut)
- 2 tablespoons apple cider vinegar
- 1 tablespoon Dijon mustard
- 1 teaspoon garlic powder
- 1 teaspoon onion powder
- 1/4 cup nutritional yeast (for a cheesy flavor)
- 1/2 teaspoon black pepper
- 1/2 cup chopped red onion
- 1/2 cup chopped celery
- 1/4 cup fresh dill, chopped (or 1 tablespoon dried dill)
- 1/2 cup plant-based bacon bits (homemade or store-bought, ensure no oil is used in preparation)
- Optional: chopped fresh parsley for garnish

Instructions:

1. Place the potatoes in a large pot and cover with water.
2. Bring to a boil, then reduce heat and simmer for about 10-15 minutes, or until the potatoes are tender but still firm.

3. Drain and let them cool slightly.
4. In a small bowl, whisk together the plant-based yogurt, apple cider vinegar, Dijon mustard, garlic powder, onion powder, nutritional yeast, and black pepper.
5. Adjust the thickness of the dressing by adding water or vegetable broth as needed to achieve a creamy consistency.
6. If using homemade plant-based bacon bits, sauté them in a non-stick pan over medium heat with a splash of water or vegetable broth until they are crispy.
7. Allow them to cool before adding them to the salad.
8. Mix the chilled potatoes, red onion, celery, dill, and vegan bacon bits in a big bowl.
9. Drizzle the sauce over the salad and carefully mix until every component is thoroughly coated.
10. Cover and refrigerate the salad for at least an hour to allow the flavors to meld together.
11. The salad can be served chilled or at room temperature.
12. Garnish with chopped fresh parsley before serving, if desired.

Roasted Vegetables

Ingredients:

- 2 medium sweet potatoes, peeled and cubed
- 2 large carrots, peeled and sliced
- 1 red bell pepper, cut into chunks
- 1 zucchini, cut into half-moons
- 1 yellow squash, cut into half-moons
- 1 red onion, cut into wedges
- 1 head of broccoli, cut into florets
- 1/4 cup low-sodium vegetable broth or water (more as needed)
- 2 teaspoons garlic powder
- 2 teaspoons onion powder
- 1 teaspoon dried thyme
- 1 teaspoon dried rosemary
- Salt and pepper to taste (optional)
- Fresh herbs for garnish (optional)

Instructions:

1. Preheat your oven to 425°F (220°C).
2. Prepare a large baking sheet by lining it with parchment paper or a silicone baking mat to prevent sticking without the use of oil.
3. Wash and chop all the vegetables into fairly uniform pieces to ensure even cooking.

4. Mix the sweet potatoes, carrots, bell pepper, zucchini, squash, onion, and broccoli in a sizable bowl.
5. Pour in the vegetable broth or water and toss until the vegetables are well coated.
6. Sprinkle the garlic powder, onion powder, dried thyme, dried rosemary, and optional salt and pepper over the vegetables.
7. Toss again to evenly distribute the seasonings.
8. Spread the seasoned vegetables out in a single layer on the prepared baking sheet. Make sure they are not overcrowded to allow for proper roasting.
9. Roast in the preheated oven for 25-35 minutes, or until the vegetables are tender and starting to caramelize around the edges.
10. Halfway through the roasting time, stir the vegetables or shake the pan to ensure even roasting.
11. If the vegetables seem dry or start to stick, you can add a little more vegetable broth or water.
12. Once roasted to your liking, remove the vegetables from the oven.
13. Taste and adjust seasoning if necessary.
14. Garnish with fresh herbs such as parsley or thyme if desired before serving.

Vegan Corn and Potato Chowder

Ingredients:

- 4 cups corn kernels (fresh or frozen)
- 2 large potatoes, diced
- 1 large sweet onion, diced
- 3 cloves garlic, minced
- 4 stalks celery, diced
- 2 carrots, peeled and diced
- 6 cups low-sodium vegetable broth
- 1 cup unsweetened almond milk or any plant-based milk
- 1 teaspoon smoked paprika
- 1 teaspoon dried thyme
- Salt and pepper to taste (optional)
- Fresh parsley for garnish

Instructions:

1. In a large pot over medium heat, add a small amount of vegetable broth to sauté the onion, garlic, celery, and carrots until they start to soften, about 5 minutes.
2. Use broth instead of oil to adhere to the starch-based diet guidelines.
3. Add the diced potatoes and the rest of the vegetable broth to the pot.
4. Bring to a simmer and cook until the potatoes are tender about 15-20 minutes.

5. Once the potatoes are soft, add the corn kernels, smoked paprika, and dried thyme to the pot.
6. Stir well to combine all the ingredients.
7. Allow the chowder to simmer for another 10 minutes for the flavors to meld together.
8. To achieve a creamy texture without using dairy or processed ingredients, take out about 2 cups of the soup (make sure to get some potatoes and corn) and blend until smooth.
9. You can use an immersion blender or a regular blender for this step.
10. Be cautious when blending hot liquids.
11. Return the blended mixture to the pot and stir well.
12. Add the plant-based milk, and adjust the seasoning with salt and pepper if desired.
13. Heat the chowder until it's warm throughout, but do not let it boil after adding the plant milk.
14. Ladle the chowder into bowls and garnish with fresh chopped parsley. Serve hot.

Apple and Onion Mix

Ingredients:

- 3 large apples (preferably a mix of sweet and tart varieties), cored and sliced
- 2 large red onions, sliced
- 1/4 cup vegetable broth or water, for sautéing
- 2 tablespoons balsamic vinegar
- 1 teaspoon dried thyme
- Salt and pepper to taste (optional)
- Fresh parsley or thyme for garnish

Instructions:

1. Start by coring and slicing the apples into thin wedges.
2. Do the same with the onions, ensuring they are sliced rather than diced to complement the apple slices in size.
3. Place a modest quantity of vegetable broth in a big non-stick skillet or pan and bring it to a simmer over medium flame.
4. Add the sliced onions and cook, stirring occasionally, until they start to soften and become translucent, about 5-7 minutes.
5. Add more broth as needed to prevent sticking.
6. To the softened onions, add the sliced apples along with the dried thyme. Stir to combine.

7. Continue to cook the apple and onion mixture for another 5-10 minutes, until the apples are tender but not mushy.
8. Keep the heat at a medium level to gently cook the apples while retaining their shape.
9. Once the apples are tender, stir in the balsamic vinegar and cook for an additional 2 minutes to allow the flavors to meld together.
10. Season with salt and pepper to taste, if desired.
11. Remove from heat and transfer to a serving dish.
12. Garnish with fresh parsley or thyme before serving.

Mixed Veggie Fried Rice

Ingredients:

- 2 cups brown rice, cooked and cooled (preferably refrigerated overnight)
- 1 cup carrots, diced
- 1 cup peas (fresh or frozen)
- 1 bell pepper, diced
- 1 cup broccoli florets, chopped
- 1/2 cup corn kernels (fresh or frozen)
- 1 large onion, diced
- 3 cloves garlic, minced
- 1/4 cup green onions, chopped
- 1/4 cup low-sodium soy sauce or tamari (ensure gluten-free if necessary)
- 1 tablespoon rice vinegar
- 1 teaspoon ground ginger
- 1/2 teaspoon black pepper
- 1/4 cup water or vegetable broth for sautéing
- Optional: chili flakes for added heat

Instructions:

1. Ensure all vegetables are washed, peeled (where necessary), and diced.
2. Have your brown rice cooked, cooled, and preferably refrigerated from the night before to achieve the best texture for fried rice.

3. Warm a small amount of water or vegetable broth in a sizable non-stick pan or wok, setting the heat to medium.
4. Incorporate the chopped onion and crushed garlic, cooking until they become transparent and emit a strong aroma, approximately 2-3 minutes.
5. Add more liquid as needed to prevent sticking.
6. To the pan, add the diced carrots, broccoli, and bell peppers.
7. Continue to cook, stirring frequently, until they start to soften, about 5 minutes.
8. Add the peas and corn to the mixture and stir well.
9. Cook for another 2-3 minutes until these vegetables are heated through but still vibrant.
10. Stir in the cold brown rice, breaking up any clumps.
11. Allow the rice to heat up in the pan, stirring occasionally.
12. Mix in the soy sauce, rice vinegar, ground ginger, and black pepper.
13. Adjust the seasonings to taste and add chili flakes if desired.

14. Once everything is well combined and the rice is heated through, finish by stirring in the chopped green onions for a fresh burst of flavor.
15. Serve the Mixed Veggie Fried Rice hot as a main dish or as a complement to other starch-based dishes.
16. It's perfect for a filling lunch or dinner, providing a balance of whole grains, vegetables, and flavors.

Vegan Potato Curry in Instapot

Ingredients:

- 2 cups brown rice, cooked and cooled (preferably refrigerated overnight)
- 1 cup carrots, diced
- 1 cup peas (fresh or frozen)
- 1 bell pepper, diced
- 1 cup broccoli florets, chopped
- 1/2 cup corn kernels (fresh or frozen)
- 1 large onion, diced
- 3 cloves garlic, minced
- 1/4 cup green onions, chopped
- 1/4 cup low-sodium soy sauce or tamari (ensure gluten-free if necessary)
- 1 tablespoon rice vinegar
- 1 teaspoon ground ginger
- 1/2 teaspoon black pepper
- 1/4 cup water or vegetable broth for sautéing
- Optional: chili flakes for added heat

Instructions:

1. Ensure all vegetables are washed, peeled (where necessary), and diced.
2. Have your brown rice cooked, cooled, and preferably refrigerated from the night before to achieve the best texture for fried rice.

3. Heat a small portion of water or vegetable broth in a broad non-stick pan or wok on medium flame.
4. Put in the chopped onion and garlic, and cook until they turn translucent and release their fragrance, taking about 2-3 minutes.
5. Add more liquid as needed to prevent sticking.
6. To the pan, add the diced carrots, broccoli, and bell peppers.
7. Continue to cook, stirring frequently, until they start to soften, about 5 minutes.
8. Add the peas and corn to the mixture and stir well.
9. Cook for another 2-3 minutes until these vegetables are heated through but still vibrant.
10. Stir in the cold brown rice, breaking up any clumps.
11. Allow the rice to heat up in the pan, stirring occasionally.
12. Mix in the soy sauce, rice vinegar, ground ginger, and black pepper.
13. Adjust the seasonings to taste and add chili flakes if desired.
14. Once everything is well combined and the rice is heated through, finish by stirring in the chopped green onions for a fresh burst of flavor.
15. Serve the Mixed Veggie Fried Rice hot as a main dish or as a complement to other starch-based dishes.
16. It's perfect for a filling lunch or dinner, providing a balance of whole grains, vegetables, and flavors.

Sweet Potato and Ginger

Ingredients:

- 2 pounds sweet potatoes, peeled and cubed
- 1 large onion, diced
- 3 cloves garlic, minced
- 2 tablespoons fresh ginger, grated
- 4 cups vegetable broth (low sodium, if preferred)
- 1 teaspoon ground cinnamon
- 1/4 teaspoon ground nutmeg
- Salt and black pepper to taste (optional)
- 1 can (about 14 oz) light coconut milk (ensure it's unsweetened for a starch-based diet)
- Juice of 1 lime
- Fresh cilantro or parsley for garnish (optional)

Instructions:

1. Begin by peeling and cubing the sweet potatoes, dicing the onion, mincing the garlic, and grating the ginger. These preparations will make the cooking process smooth and efficient.
2. In a large pot, add a small amount of water or vegetable broth over medium heat.
3. Incorporate the chopped onion, crushed garlic, and shredded ginger.
4. Cook until the onion is translucent and the mixture is fragrant about 5 minutes.

5. Stir occasionally and add more liquid as needed to prevent sticking.
6. To the pot, add the cubed sweet potatoes, vegetable broth, ground cinnamon, and ground nutmeg.
7. Stir well to combine all the ingredients. Bring the mixture to a boil, then reduce the heat to low, cover, and simmer until the sweet potatoes are tender, about 20-25 minutes.
8. After the sweet potatoes have become tender and thoroughly cooked, take the pot off the stove.
9. Using an immersion blender, blend the soup directly in the pot until smooth and creamy.
10. Alternatively, you can carefully transfer the soup to a blender, blend until smooth, and then return it to the pot. Be cautious when blending hot liquids.
11. Stir in the light coconut milk and the juice of one lime into the blended soup.
12. Place the pot back on low heat to warm through, stirring well.
13. Taste and adjust seasoning with salt and black pepper, if desired.
14. Ladle the Sweet Potato and Ginger Soup into bowls.
15. Garnish with fresh cilantro or parsley leaves for a touch of color and added flavor.

16. Serve the soup warm as a nourishing starter or as a main dish.
17. It's delightful on its own or paired with a side of whole-grain bread for dipping.

Rice and Peas

Ingredients:

- 2 cups long-grain brown rice
- 1 cup dried kidney beans or pigeon peas, soaked overnight and drained
- 4 cups water (for cooking beans)
- 3 cups homemade coconut milk (ensure it's unsweetened and made from fresh or unsweetened shredded coconut)
- 2 green onions, chopped
- 2 cloves garlic, minced
- 1 Scotch bonnet pepper (whole, for flavor, or removed depending on spice preference)
- 2 sprigs of fresh thyme or 1 teaspoon dried thyme
- 3 whole allspice berries (pimento seeds)
- Salt to taste (optional, and minimal if used)

Instructions:

1. In a large pot, add the soaked and drained kidney beans or pigeon peas along with 4 cups of water.
2. Bring to a boil, then reduce heat, cover, and simmer until the beans are tender but not falling apart, about 1-2 hours depending on the type of bean and whether they were pre-soaked.
3. Once the beans are cooked, add the homemade coconut milk, green onions, minced garlic, whole

Scotch bonnet pepper, thyme, allspice berries, and salt (if using) to the pot.
4. Rinse the brown rice under cold water and then add it to the pot.
5. Bring the mixture to a boil, then reduce the heat to low, cover, and simmer until the rice is tender and the liquid has been absorbed about 40-50 minutes.
6. Check occasionally to ensure the rice doesn't stick to the bottom of the pot.
7. Once the rice is cooked, remove the pot from the heat.
8. Carefully remove the Scotch bonnet pepper (if it was left whole), thyme sprigs, and allspice berries.
9. Fluff the rice with a fork to mix the peas evenly throughout.
10. Serve the Rice and Peas hot as a delicious and nutritious side dish.
11. It pairs wonderfully with other plant-based dishes, making for a complete and satisfying meal.

Baked Potato

Ingredients:

- 4 large russet potatoes, scrubbed clean
- Toppings (choose based on your preference):
- Chopped green onions or chives
- Salsa (ensure it's oil-free and low in sugar)
- Steamed broccoli florets
- Black beans, rinsed and drained
- Homemade cashew cheese sauce (made from blended cashews, nutritional yeast, garlic powder, onion powder, and a bit of water for consistency)
- Avocado slices or guacamole (in moderation due to high-fat content)
- A sprinkle of nutritional yeast for a cheesy flavor

Instructions:

1. Preheat your oven to 425°F (220°C). While the oven is heating, pierce each potato several times with a fork.
2. This allows steam to escape and prevents the potatoes from bursting in the oven.
3. Place the potatoes directly on the middle rack of your oven (you can place a baking sheet on the lower rack to catch any drippings).
4. Bake for about 45-60 minutes, or until the potatoes are tender inside when pierced with a fork.

5. While the potatoes are baking, prepare your chosen toppings.
6. If you're using vegetables, like broccoli, steam them until just tender.
7. For beans, ensure they're well-rinsed and heated through.
8. If making a cashew cheese sauce, blend the ingredients until smooth, adjusting the consistency with a little water as needed.
9. After the potatoes are finished cooking, take them out of the oven and allow them to cool down for a short period.
10. Next, gently cut each potato open along its length. Watch out for the steam!
11. Fluff the insides of the potatoes with a fork to make room for your toppings.
12. Add your chosen toppings to each potato.
13. There's no right or wrong way to do this—mix and match flavors according to your taste preferences!
14. Serve your customized baked potatoes hot.
15. Enjoy the hearty, comforting flavors knowing you're adhering to your starch-based dietary preferences.

Conclusion

The Starch-Based Diet is a good way to start converting to a healthier and more reliable diet, especially for those who need it for health reasons. As studies show, and even based on the evidence seen on Asians, the Starch-Based Diet can be a good option for anyone who wants to get rid of junk foods and unhealthy lifestyles they have gotten used to.

Developed after seeing how this greatly affected generations of Asian immigrants after living in the US, Dr. McDougall conducted intensive research on how starchy food greatly benefitted the older generation but not the younger ones.

Generally, starchy foods are normally part of one's regular diet and must be consumed, at least weekly, to keep a healthy balanced diet. However, a restricted starch-based diet will also be beneficial for those who must eliminate specific food items from their diet due to allergies, intolerance, or sensitivities.

A starch-based diet mainly includes bread, pasta, cereals, potatoes, grains, and rice. These food options are great for vegetarians. This diet is also rich in minerals and nutrients essential for the body to function well. These include fiber, iron, calcium, and B vitamins.

Just like any diet, there are pros and cons to this one as well. Because this is restrictive in a way, one may experience nutrient deficiency. This is why guidance from a health expert is important when starting this diet.

FAQs

What is a Starch-Based Diet?

It's a diet mainly consisting of starchy food items such as bread, corn, pasta potatoes, and lentils, to name a few. It was developed by John McDougall, MD after studying the health decline of generations of Asian-American immigrants. The younger generation's health declined drastically as compared to their elders after fully embracing the all-American diet.

What are the benefits of a Starch-Based Diet?

It's mainly vegan-friendly and focuses on getting rid of unhealthy food options. A starch-based diet is also rich in fiber, B vitamins, iron, and calcium.

How would a starch-based diet affect one's health?

Starchy foods are part of a recommended food diet grouped into five. As they are rich in fiber and B vitamins at least, they are mainly important to promote good health digestion.

Can I get enough protein on a starch-based diet?

Yes, you can obtain sufficient protein on a starch-based diet. Many starch-rich foods, especially beans, lentils, and whole grains, are good sources of protein. By consuming a variety of plant-based foods and ensuring adequate calorie intake, most people can meet their protein needs without difficulty.

It's important to include a diverse range of starches and other plant-based foods to ensure a comprehensive nutrient profile.

Is a starch-based diet expensive to follow?

A starch-based diet can be very economical. Starch-rich foods like potatoes, rice, and beans are often less expensive than meat and dairy products. By focusing on these staples along with seasonal fruits and vegetables, one can maintain a cost-effective, healthy diet. Planning meals and purchasing whole foods in bulk can further reduce expenses.

Will I feel hungry all the time on a starch-based diet?

Contrary to expectations, a starch-based diet can keep you full and satisfied. Starches are complex carbs that digest slowly, offering steady energy and curbing hunger. The fiber in these foods also helps you feel full. Transitioning from processed foods may require adjustment, but many feel more satisfied with this diet.

Are there any foods strictly off-limits on a starch-based diet?

A starch-based diet focuses on whole, plant-based foods while limiting animal products, processed foods, sugars, and oils. Emphasize eating foods in their natural state for optimal nutrients and health benefits. Tailor the diet to suit your needs and preferences for a sustainable and enjoyable experience.

How can I start a starch-based diet if I'm used to eating a lot of meat and dairy?

Transitioning to a starch-based diet from a meat and dairy-heavy one is a big change. Start by adding more starch-rich plant foods to your meals while cutting back on meat and dairy. Try plant-based options, and new recipes, and educate yourself on nutrition for a smoother transition. Take it step by step, adjusting the diet to fit your lifestyle and tastes.

References and Helpful Links

7 Ways to Optimal health with a Starch-Based Diet | Dr. McDougall. (2024, January 18). Dr. McDougall. https://www.drmcdougall.com/education/nutrition/7-ways-to-optimal-health-and-well-being-with-a-starch-based-diet/

Ashokan, M. (2019, April 11). Simple Vs Complex Carbs: Which One Is Better For Quick Weight Loss? Health. Retrieved August 19, 2020 from https://www.ndtv.com/health/simple-vs-complex-carbs-which-one-is-better-for-quick-weight-loss-2021317.

Blue Zones. (2016, November). Is Sugar Really Making Us Fat? Retrieved August 19, 2020, from https://www.bluezones.com/2016/11/sugar-isnt-making-you-fat/.

Bourassa, L. (2020, July 13). What Is the Starch Solution? Very Well Fit. Retrieved August 19, 2020, from https://www.verywellfit.com/the-starch-solution-diet-4771538.

Chang, S. (2020). Back to Basics: All About MyPlate Food Groups. Usda.gov. https://www.usda.gov/media/blog/2017/09/26/back-basics-all-about-myplate-food-groups.

Dr. McDougall's Health & Medical Center | Dr. McDougall. (2024,

Editorial Staff Woman's World. (2018, November 20). This Carb-Friendly Cleanse Mimics the Effects of Gastric Bypass. Woman's World. Retrieved August 221, 2020 from https://www.womansworld.com/posts/health/resistant-starch-diet-143267.

Harvard School of Public Health. (2018, June 6). Fiber. The Nutrition Source; The President and Fellows of Harvard College. https://www.hsph.harvard.edu/nutritionsource/carbohydrates/fiber/.

Higgins, J. A. (2014). Resistant Starch and Energy Balance: Impact on Weight Loss and Maintenance. Critical Reviews in Food Science and Nutrition, 54(9), 1158–1166. https://doi.org/10.1080/10408398.2011.629352.

John, R., & Ting, T. (2016). Starch-Based Diet and Type 2 Diabetes. Journal of Health Disparities Research and Practice, 9(5). https://digitalscholarship.unlv.edu/jhdrp/vol9/iss5/40/.

John, R., Jr, & Ting, T. Y. (n.d.). Starch-Based diet and Type 2 diabetes. Digital Scholarship@UNLV. https://digitalscholarship.unlv.edu/jhdrp/vol9/iss5/40/#:~:text=The%20starch%20based%20diet%20was,his%20patients%20reverse%20their%20diabetes.

Kahn, J. (2015, September 29). Why This Doctor Wants You To Consider A Starch-Based Diet, Mindbodygreen. Retrieved August 20, 2020, from https://www.mindbodygreen.com/0-21794/why-this-doctor-wants-you-to-consider-a-starchbased-diet.html.

Laurence, E. (2018, August 22). Pretty Much Every Keto No-No Is a Yes on This Diet. Healthy Eating Plans. Retrieved August 19, 2020, from https://www.wellandgood.com/starch-diet-guidelines/.

McDougall, J. (2023). The role of a starch-based diet in solving existential challenges for the 21st century. Frontiers in Nutrition, 10, 1260455. https://doi.org/10.3389/fnut.2023.1260455.

Montouri, N. (2018, July 22). Podcast #41: The Starch Based Diet with Dr. John McDougall. Ordinary Vegan. Retrieved August 20, 2020 from https://ordinaryvegan.net/starch-based-diet-john-mcdougall/.

Muinos, L. (2022, November 4). What is the starch Solution diet? Verywell Fit. https://www.verywellfit.com/the-starch-solution-diet-4771538

NHS. (2023, March 15). Starchy foods and carbohydrates. Nhs.uk. https://www.nhs.uk/live-well/eat-well/food-types/starchy-foods-and-carbohydrates/.

Nidirect. (2023, February 20). Starchy foods. Nidirect. https://www.nidirect.gov.uk/articles/starchy-foods#:~:text=Potatoes%2C%20bread%2C%20rice%2C%20pasta,half%20the%20calories%20of%20fat.

Our Story. (n.d.). Dr. McDougall. https://www.drmcdougall.com/our-story/.

Plant-Based Diets. (2014, October 22). What to Eat on A Plant-Based Diet (McDougall Starch Version). Fanatic Cook. Retrieved August 20, 2020 from https://fanaticcook.com/2014/10/22/what-to-eat-on-a-plant-based-diet-mcdougall-starch-version/.

Popkin, B., Adair, L., Ng, S.W. (2012, January). NOW AND THEN: The Global Nutrition Transition: The Pandemic of Obesity in Developing Countries. Department of Nutrition and Carolina Population Center, University of North Carolina at Chapel Hill. Retrieved August 221, 2020 from https://www.ncbi.nlm.nih.gov/pmc/articles/PMC3257829/#R13.

Starch Solution Meal Planner & Recipes | Dr. McDougall. (2022, January 3). Dr. McDougall. https://www.drmcdougall.com/education/free-mcdougall-program/10-day-meal-plan/

Starch Solution: Eat Carbs and Lose Weight. (n.d.). Www.freedieting.com. Retrieved January 4, 2024, from https://www.freedieting.com/starch-solution.

Starchy foods - British Nutrition Foundation. (n.d.). Www.nutrition.org.uk. https://www.nutrition.org.uk/healthy-sustainable-diets/starchy-foods-sugar-and-fibre/starchy-foods/?level=Consumer.

Starchy foods | nidirect. (2015, November 26). Www.nidirect.gov.uk. https://www.nidirect.gov.uk/articles/starchy-foods.

The eatwell guide and resources | food standards agency. (n.d.). Retrieved January 5, 2024, from https://www.food.gov.uk/business-guidance/the-eatwell-guide-and-resources.

Thriving on Plants. (n.d.). What are Starch-Based Vegan Diets? Plant-Based Diets. Retrieved August 19, 2020, from https://www.thrivingonplants.com/starch-based-vegan-diets/.

U.S. Department of Health & Human Services. (2015). Dietary Guidelines for Americans2025-2020 Eight Edition. Retrieved August 20, 2020, from https://health.gov/our-work/food-nutrition/2015-2020-dietary-guidelines/guidelines/.

U.S. Department of Health & Human Services. (January 26, 2017) Importance of Good Nutrition, Content created by President's Council on Sports, Fitness & Nutrition. Retrieved August 19, 2020, from https://www.hhs.gov/fitness/eat-healthy/importance-of-good-nutrition/index.html.

United Nations. (n.d.). LIFESTYLE DISEASES: An economic burden on the health services | United Nations. https://www.un.org/en/chronicle/article/lifestyle-diseases-economic-burden-health-services#:~:text=Lifestyle%20diseases%20share%20risk%20factors,metabolic%20syndrome%2C%20chronic%20obstructive%20pulmonary

WebMD Editorial Contributors. (2020, November 3). Foods high in starch. WebMD. https://www.webmd.com/diet/foods-high-in-starch

Website, N. (2023, March 20). Starchy foods and carbohydrates. nhs.uk. https://www.nhs.uk/live-well/eat-well/food-types/starchy-foods-and-carbohydrates/

www.ingramcontent.com/pod-product-compliance
Lightning Source LLC
LaVergne TN
LVHW010427070526
838199LV00066B/5948